This Notebook belongs to

....

www.ingramcontent.com/pod-product-compliance
Lightning Source LLC
Chambersburg PA
CBHW072211280526
45788CB00002B/974
* 9 7 8 1 0 9 1 1 4 6 1 8 1 *